THE YOGA
HANDBOOK
ADVANCED YOGA POSES

OPINDER CHAGGAR

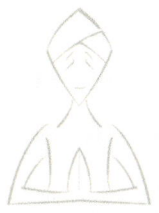

Copyright (c) 2018 Opinder Chaggar
All rights reserved
ISBN: 9781718174757

WWW.YOGASIMRAN.NET

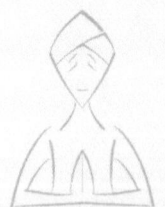

Yoga is a physical exercise great for health however always consult your doctor before doing any physical activities.

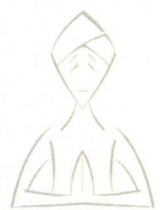

Dedicated to
my Mother and Father
Darshan Kaur Chaggar
and
Balbir Singh Chaggar

For their continued love and support,
whatever path I took

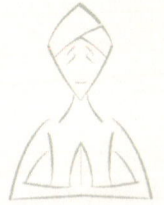

Contents

The Yoga Handbook - Introduction	6
What Is Yoga?	7
Natarajasana (Lord of the Dance Pose)	8
Eka pada urdhva dhanurasana (one-legged wheel pose)	10
Kapotasana (One Legged King Pigeon Pose)	12
Karnapidasana Utkatasana (Ear Pressure Pose)	14
Surya Namaskārāsana (Sun Salutation Pose)	16
Baddha Samakonasana (Bound Equal Angle Pose)	18
Tittibhasana (Firefly Pose)	20
Paschimottanasana (Seated Forward Bend or Intense Dorsal Stretch)	22
Mukhottanasana (Reverse Facing Intense Stretch Pose)	24
Eka Pada Paripurna Vrschikasana is an Asana (One Legged Stretched Out Scorpion Pose)	26
Karnapidasana Utkatasana (Ear Pressure Pose)	28
Eka pada urdhva dhanurasana (one-legged wheel pose)	30
Naam Simran Chant Mantra	32

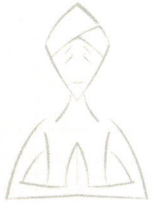

The Yoga Handbook
Introduction

Thank you so much for choosing to purchase my book,
'The Yoga Handbook'

My name is Opinder Chaggar
I am a student of yoga and a full time 3D Animator and Artist.

My love for drawing led me to think how I could share
my positive experiences through Yoga and Meditation (Simran).
Since I love to draw I thought what better way to show my basic
morning routine by drawing ten effective poses that have helped
me feel energised and ready on a daily basis.

(Note you don't have to do these in the morning,
you can fit them whenever they suit your schedule.)
Although the handbook states hold poses for 10-12 breaths.
Do what suits you at the start and build from there. See how you
feel and adjust accordingly.

You could hold for minutes too but
I just want to emphasise the importance of the breath (Pranas)
too. Focusing on breathing is the most important aspect,
I would say be conscious of your breath.

Creating this habit will see growth
in your daily mood and positive attitude,
especially the end part Meditation (Simran). Apply this into
your morning routine everyday finishing with powerful Meditation
at the end and you'll awaken your chakras.

Thank you once again for purchasing
'The Yoga Handbook' I have thoroughly
enjoyed the creative process,
I hope you have as much fun with these poses
as I did drawing them!

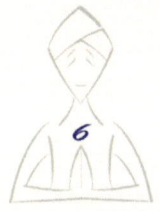

What Is Yoga?

Katha Upanishad
"When the five senses, along with the mind, remain still and the intellect is not active, that is known as the highest state. They consider yoga to be firm restraint of the senses. Then one becomes un-distracted for yoga is the arising and the passing away"

Bhagavad Gita
"Yoga is said to be equanimity"
"Yoga is skill in action"
"Know that which is called yoga to be separation from contact with suffering"

Yogacarabhumi – Sravakabhumi
"Yoga is fourfold: faith, aspiration, perseverance and means"

Yoga Sutras of Patanjali
"Yoga is the suppression of the activities of the mind"

Vaisesika sutra
"Pleasure and suffering arise as a result of the drawing together of the sense organs, the mind and objects. When that does not happen because the mind is in the self, there is no pleasure or suffering for one who is embodied. That is yoga"

Kaundinya's Pancarthabhasya on the Pasupatasutra
"In this system, yoga is the union of the self"

Linga Purana
"By the word 'yoga' is meant nirvana"

Brahmasutra-bhasya of Adi Shankara
"It is said in the treatises on yoga: 'Yoga is the means of perceiving reality.'"

Guru Nanak
"Conquer your mind and conquer the world"

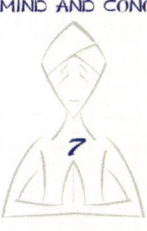

Benefits Of Natarajasana (Lord of the Dance Pose)

Assists in – losing weight as you tend to burn calories during practice

Strengthens and stretches – your ankles, legs, thighs, chest, abdomen, thorax, and hips

Develops – greater flexibility in your spine shoulders, and hamstrings

Improves – your balance

Acts as – a great stress buster, calming your mind

Greatly improves – your digestive system

Concentration – increasing in intensity

Invigoration – is felt after practicing this posture, since it activates your entire body

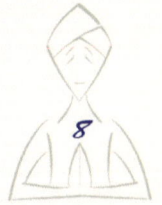

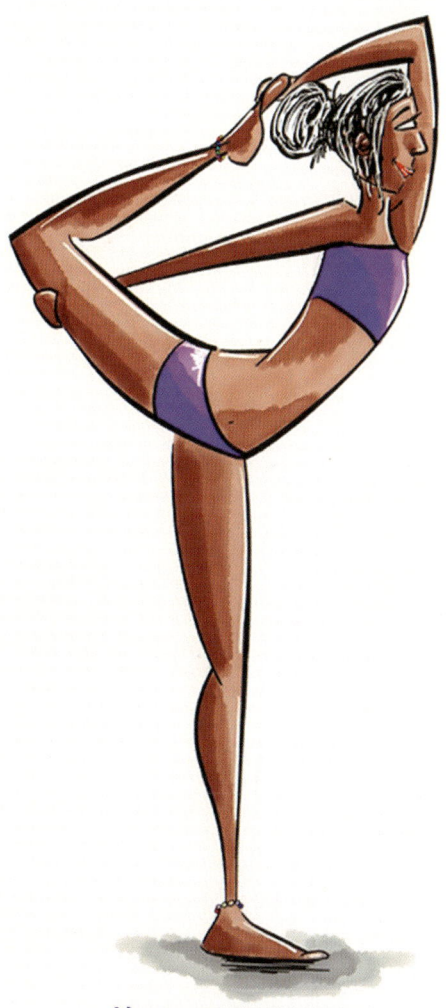

NATARAJASANA
(LORD OF THE DANCE POSE)

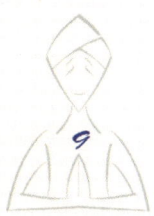

Benefits Of
Eka Pada Urdhva Dhanurasana
(One-Legged Wheel Pose)

Increases - feelings of self-love and compassion

Energizes - both body and mind

Increases - spinal flexibility

Soothes - anxiety and depression

Promotes - calm and serenity

Increases - mental alertness

Improves - balance

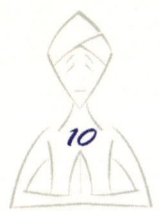

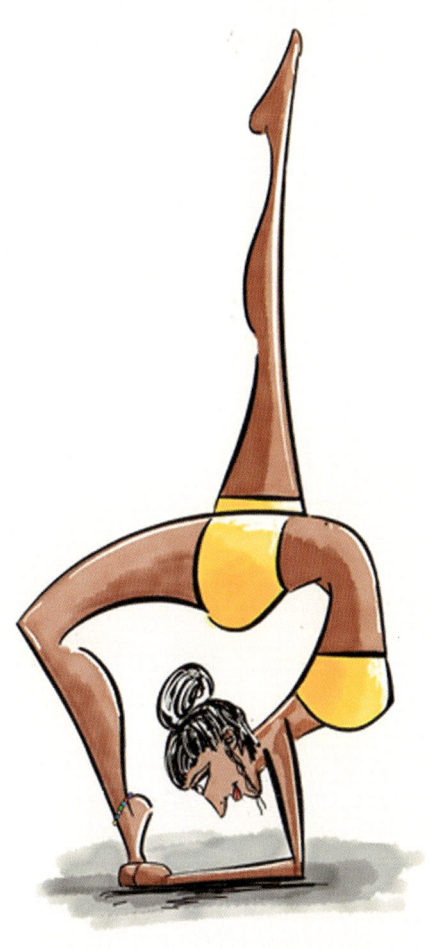

Eka pada urdhva dhanurasana
(One-legged wheel pose)

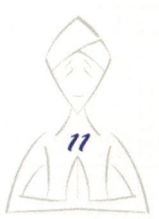

Benefits Of KAPOTASANA
(One Legged King Pigeon Pose)

Stretches and strengthens - the joints and muscles in your legs

Helps to reduce - stiffness in the back and hips

Balances - the blood pressure and also

Reduces - the effects of chronic diseases

Releases - stress and calms the mind and the body

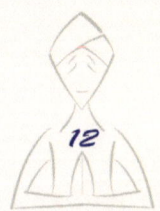

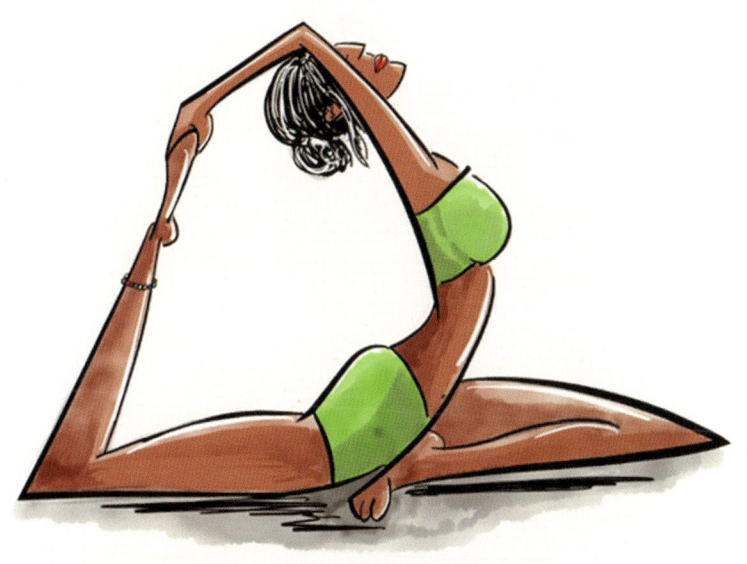

KAPOTASANA
(One Legged King Pigeon Pose)

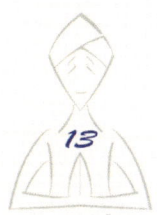

Benefits Of Karnapidasana Utkatasana (Ear Pressure Pose)

Stretches - and strengthens your back bone

Gives strength - to the lungs

Beneficial for - asthma patients

Stimulates - the abdominal organs, and thyroid gland

Stretches - the shoulders and spine

Controls – hypertension

Reduces - the symptoms of menopause

Helps to alleviate - fatigue, stress, insomnia, and negative symptoms of menopause

Helpful in - backache, infertility, sinusitis

Gives - deeper spinal flexion and an intense stretch of the hips

Good for - internal abdominal massage to the organs

Tones - the buttocks, hips and thighs during stretching the shoulders and neck

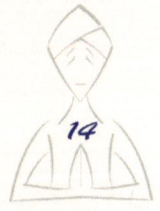

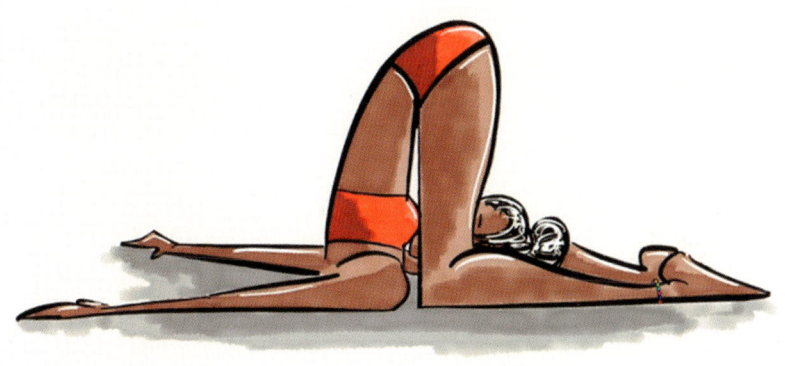

Karnapidasana Utkatasana
(Ear Pressure Pose)

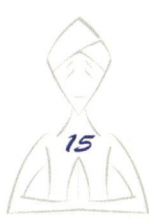

Benefits Of Surya Namaskārāsana (Sun Salutation Pose)

Helps – lose weight

Helps strengthen – muscles and joints

Gives – glowing skin

Ensures – a better functioning digestive system

Helps – cope with insomnia

Ensures – regular menstrual cycle

Brings down – blood sugar levels

Keeps – anxiety at bay

Helps – detox

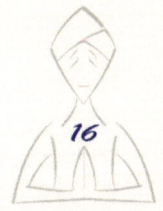

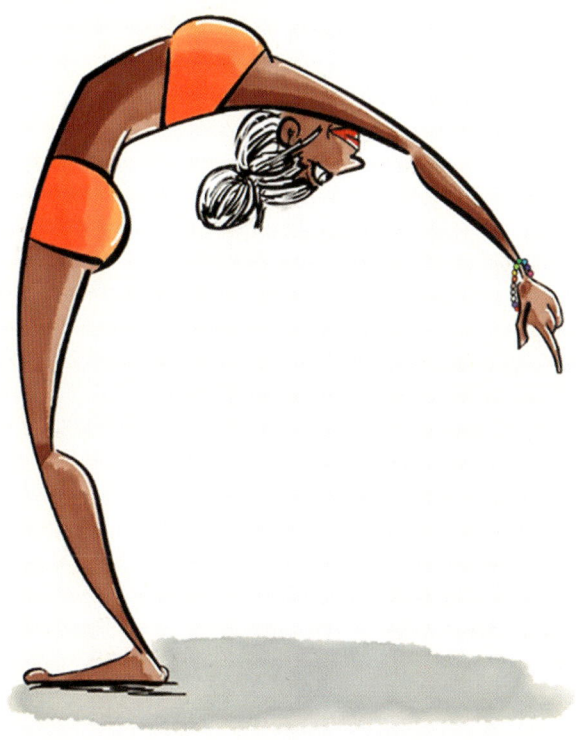

Surya Namaskārāsana
(Sun Salutation Pose)

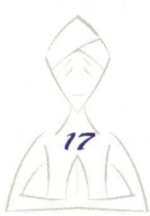

Benefits Of Baddha Samakonasana (Bound Equal Angle Pose)

Calms – the mind

Stretches – the hamstrings, groins, hips and spine

Strengthens – the back

Stimulates – the abdominal organs

Recommended for – people with sciatic pain and arthritis

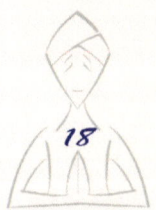

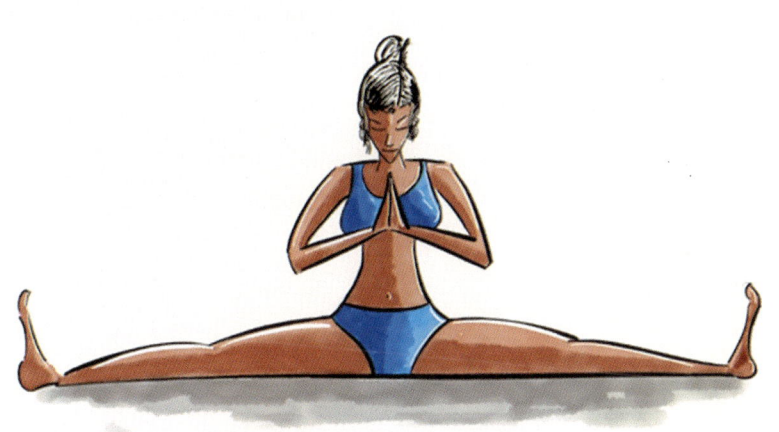

Baddha Samakonasana
(Bound Equal Angle Pose)

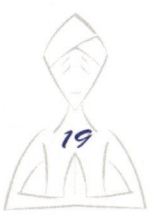

Benefits Of Tittibhasana (Firefly Pose)

Stretches - the inner groins and back torso

Strengthens - the arms and wrists

Tones - the belly

Improves - sense of balance

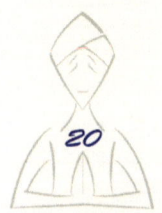

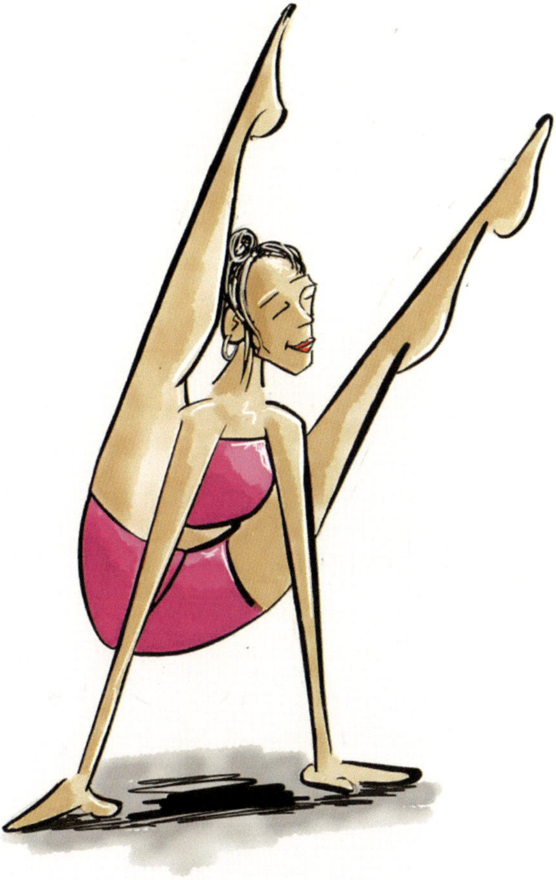

Tittibhasana
(Firefly Pose)

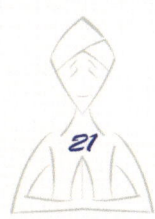

Benefits Of Paschimottanasana (Seated Forward Bend or Intense Dorsal Stretch)

Strengthens - the abdominals, hip flexors and lower back

Lengthens - the spine

Stimulates - the internal organs, particularly the liver, kidneys and reproductive organs

Improves — digestion

Calms - the mind and reduces stress

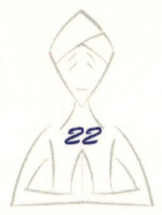

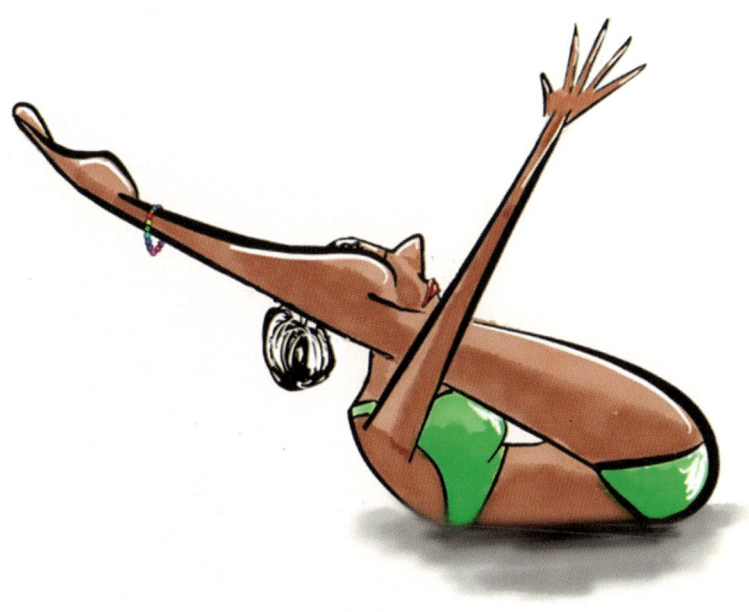

Paschimottanasana
(Seated Forward Bend
or
Intense Dorsal Stretch)

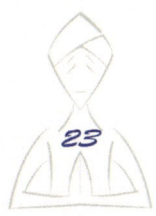

Benefits Of Mukhottanasana (Reverse Facing Intense Stretch Pose)

Stretches – The Abdominal Muscles

Increase – Spinal Flexibility

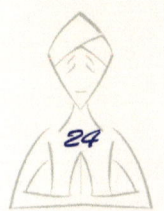

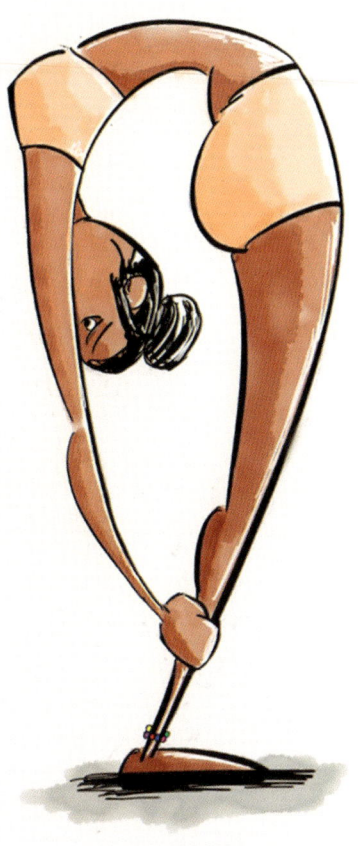

**MUKHOTTANASANA
(REVERSE FACING INTENSE STRETCH POSE)**

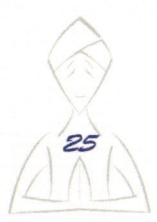

Benefits Of Eka Pada Paripurna Vrschikasana is an Asana (One Legged Stretched Out Scorpion Pose)

Creates - a sense of balance

Strengthens - the upper back and shoulders

Strengthens - the core

Stretches - the abdominals and front of the thighs

Promotes - spinal flexibility

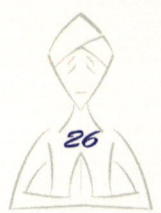

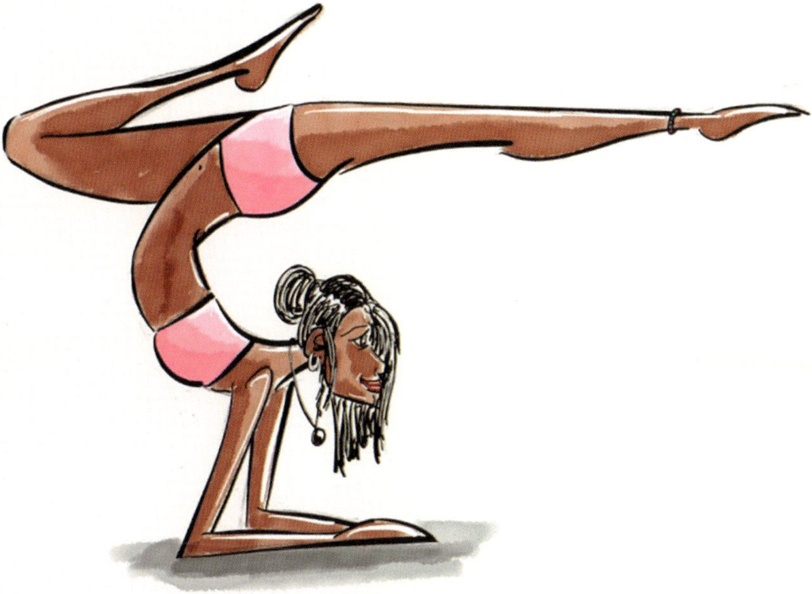

Eka Pada Paripurna Vrschikasana is an Asana (One Legged Stretched Out Scorpion Pose)

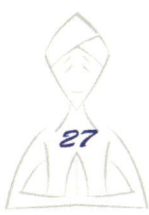

Benefits Of Karnapidasana Utkatasana (Ear Pressure Pose)

Stretches - and strengthens your back bone

Gives strength - to the lungs

Beneficial for - asthma patients

Stimulates - the abdominal organs, and thyroid gland

Stretches - the shoulders and spine

Controls - hypertension

Reduces - the symptoms of menopause

Helps to alleviate - fatigue, stress, insomnia, and negative symptoms of menopause

Helpful in - backache, infertility, sinusitis

Gives - deeper spinal flexion and an intense stretch of the hips

Good for - internal abdominal massage to the organs

Tones - the buttocks, hips and thighs during stretching the shoulders and neck

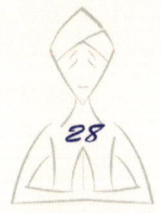

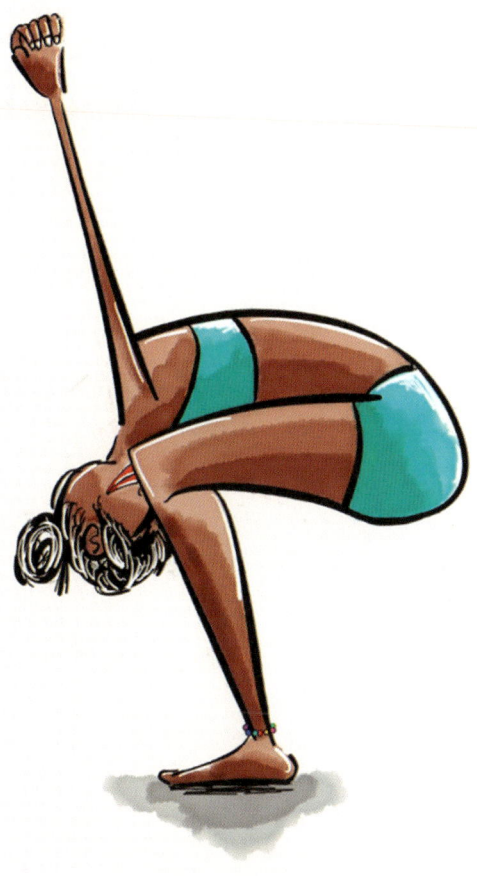

Karnapidasana Utkatasana
(Ear Pressure Pose)

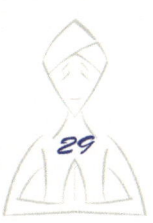

Benefits Of Eka Pada Urdhva Dhanurasana (One-Legged Wheel Pose)

Stretches - and strengthens your back bone

Increases - feelings of self-love and compassion

Energizes - both body and mind

Increases - spinal flexibility

Soothes - anxiety and depression

Promotes - calm and serenity

Increases - mental alertness

Improves - balance

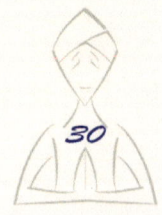

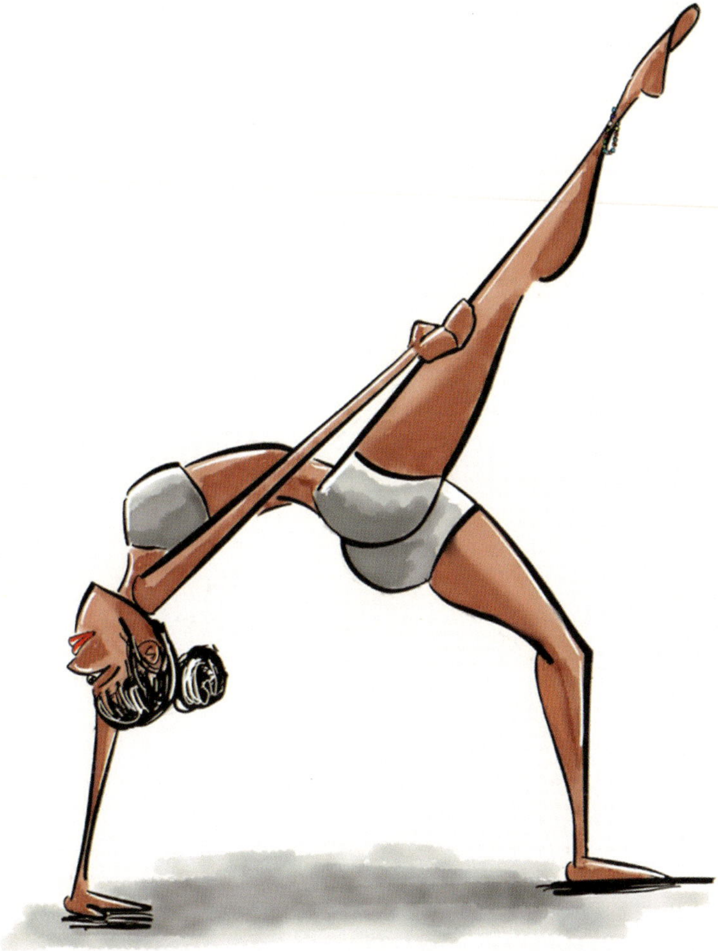

Eka pada urdhva dhanurasana
(One-legged wheel pose)

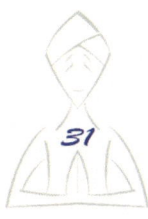

Benefits of Naam Simran

Chant Mantra 'Waheguru'

(Or find a mantra you like and chant it, find a sound that you can chant that will help clear your mind. In this practice you are trying to reduce mind chatter by listening to the sound you are chanting and concentrating on it or if you find it hard to concentrate then focus on your breathing.)

SIMRAN MEANING

Recommeneded early morning
in the ambrosial necter hours
3am – 6am (Amrit Vela)
though can be done anytime
that suits you

Simran means the remembrance
of the soul within,
the creative primal energy
inside each living being.
Tap in to become the best you

THE BENEFITS

Winning – the mind
Makes us – fearless
Humbleness no desires
No worries
Smoothness in daily life
Divine qualities
No illusions or delusions (Maya)
Contentment

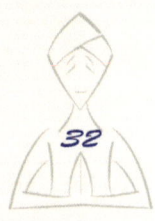

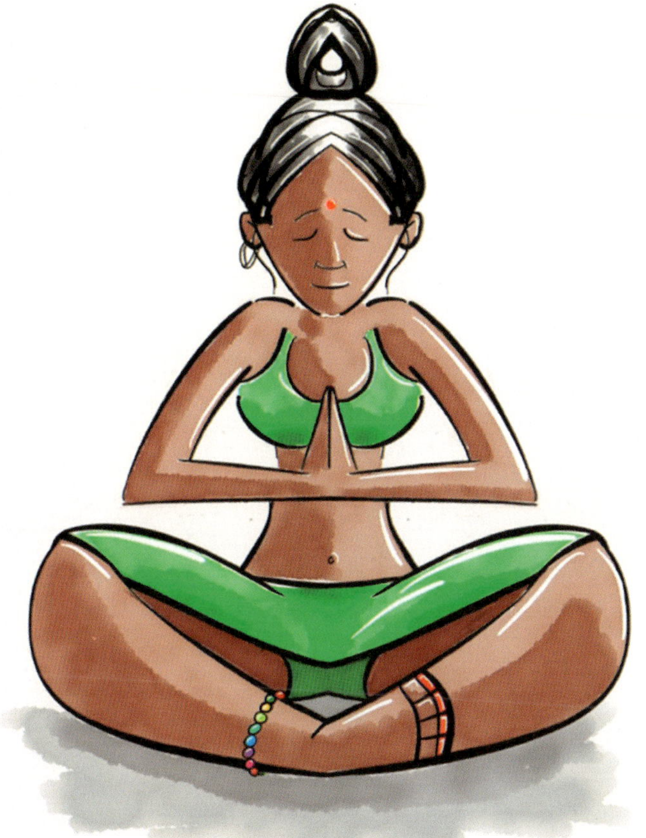

**Naam Simran
Chant Mantra**

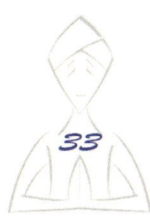

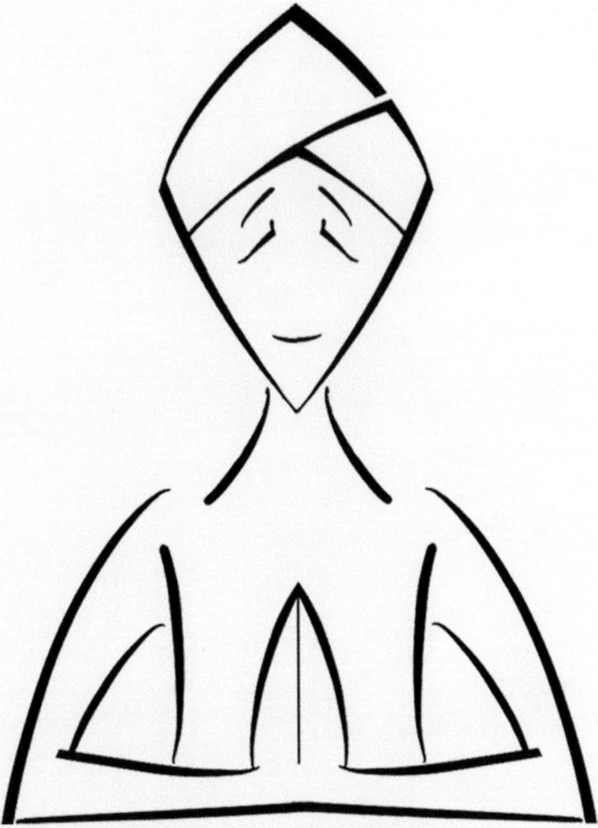

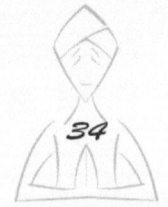

Printed in Great Britain
by Amazon